Low Carb:
20 Fast and Easy Low Carb Diet Recipes

Table of Contents

Introduction
FREE BONUS AT THE END OF THIS BOOK!

I want to thank you and congratulate you for downloading the book, *"Weight Loss Recipes: 20 Fast and Easy Low Carb Diet Recipes"*.

This book contains proven steps and strategies on how to create delicious low carb diet recipes that can help you lose weight.

Out of low carb recipe ideas? Whether you are a beginner who is trying out low carb recipes for the first time or an old timer who is looking for new dishes to enjoy, this book will be of tremendous help for you! It contains recipes for 20 mouthwatering meals that you can prepare for yourself and your family.

Each serving of the dishes in this book contains less than 10 grams of carbohydrates so you can enjoy them without worrying about your carbohydrate intake. Furthermore, you don't have to allot too much of your time in creating the dishes since each one of them does not take more than 30 minutes to cook!

In addition, you will find a bonus chapter containing recipes for low carb desserts and snacks that can help you in satisfying your sweet cravings guilt-free.

Thanks again for downloading this book, I hope you enjoy it!

Chapter 1 - The Low Carb Diet

It is not unusual for people to blame the calories in their food for every pound that they gain. As a result, many adopt a low calorie diet with the hopes of losing weight and staying healthy.

However, what they do not know is that they are only setting themselves up for failure. Low calorie food products such as cereals, pasta, and bread usually contain high amounts of unhealthy carbohydrates that prevent them from achieving their weight loss goals.

Unhealthy carbohydrates can't keep you full for long periods of time. As a result, you would end up consuming more carbohydrates in your efforts to satisfy your hunger. Some of these will be burned by your body as energy but others will be unused and stored in your body as fat. This is why it is not surprising that you are still gaining weight despite being in a low calorie diet.

Instead of obsessing over your calorie intake, it would be best to limit the amount of carbohydrates that you eat in order to lose those unwanted pounds. Furthermore, a low carb diet has numerous health benefits that can help improve your overall well-being.

Benefits of a Low Carb Diet

The main benefits of adopting a low carb diet are the following:

  ☐ A low carb diet can help you reduce your food consumption

Dishes with low amounts of carbohydrates usually contain high amounts of protein and fat. This can help you feel full for a longer period of time, thus, decreasing your food intake. In addition, this can help you stick to your diet as you won't frequently feel hungry.

  ☐ A low carb diet can help you lose more weight.

Once you cut back on your carbohydrate intake, your body will be forced to convert its stored fat into energy. Furthermore, it can decrease your blood insulin levels which will eventually cause the body to get rid of excess water resulting to further weight loss.

  ☐ A low carb diet can help reduce the risk of certain illnesses.

Carbohydrate consumption can increase the levels of triglycerides or fat molecules in your blood and make you more susceptible to heart diseases and other related illnesses. Restricting the amount of carbohydrates that you eat can help you to keep it at its normal levels and reduce the risk of cardiovascular diseases.

Low carb diet can also reduce sugar and insulin levels in your blood which can help you avoid Type 2 diabetes. It also lowers down blood pressure which can reduce the risk of numerous diseases such as stroke, hypertension and kidney failure.

Furthermore, it can increase the amount of good cholesterol in your body and, at the same time, improve the pattern of bad cholesterol.

Chapter 2 - Egg Dishes

1. Creamy Baked Eggs

Preparation Time: 5 minutes

Cook Time: 15 minutes

Number of Servings: 4

Ingredients:

1 tablespoon butter, unsalted and softened

1 tablespoon parsley, chopped

8 tablespoons heavy cream

8 eggs

Black pepper

Kosher salt

Preparation:

a. Preheat oven to 425 degrees.

b. Lightly grease 4-oz. ramekins using butter.

c. Spread 2 tablespoons of cream at the bottom of each ramekin.

d. Place 2 eggs on top of the cream in each ramekin. Season to taste.

e. Put the ramekins in the oven and let them cook for about 12 minutes.

f. Once egg whites are set, remove from the oven and garnish with parsley. This dish is best served with toast.

Nutritional Information:

Each serving contains 271 calories, 74 milligrams of calcium, 24 grams of fat, 2 milligrams of iron, 12 grams of saturated fat, 1 gram of sugar, 471 milligrams of cholesterol, 2 grams of carbohydrates, 392 milligrams of sodium and 13 grams of protein.

2. Greek Frittata

Preparation Time: 10 minutes

Cook Time: 30 minutes

Number of Servings: 4

Ingredients:

3 tablespoons olive oil

8 oz. feta, crumbled

10 eggs

5 oz. baby spinach

4 scallions, sliced thinly

2 teaspoons kosher salt

1 pint grape tomatoes, halved

½ teaspoon black pepper

Preparation:

a. Preheat oven to 350 degrees.

b. Pour olive oil in a 2-quart casserole and heat it in the oven for about 5 minutes.

c. In the meantime, beat the eggs in a bowl. Season to taste.

d. Add spinach, scallions and tomatoes into the egg mixture. Mix well.

e. Gently fold the feta in the egg mixture.

f. Remove the casserole from the oven and pour the egg mixture into it.

g. Place the casserole with the egg mixture back in the oven and allow it to bake for 30 minutes.

Nutritional Information:

Each serving contains 461 calories, 2 grams of fiber, 35 grams of fat, 5 grams of sugar, 4 grams of saturated fat, 8 grams of carbohydrates, 579 milligrams of cholesterol, 26 grams of protein and 1,868 milligrams of sodium.

3. Shirred Eggs

Preparation Time: 10 minutes

Cook Time: 20 minutes

Number of Servings: 8

Ingredients:

1 tablespoon olive oil

¼ cup heavy cream

1 teaspoon red wine vinegar

8 eggs

6 slices bread, whole grain

1 ½ cups tomatoes, chopped

¼ lb. prosciutto

2 tablespoons chives, chopped

Preparation:

a. Preheat oven to 375 degrees.

b. Place olive oil, tomatoes, vinegar and 1 tablespoon of chives in the bowl and mix well.

c. Place the bread in a single layer at the bottom of a 13" by 9" baking dish.

d. Distribute the tomato mixture and prosciutto on top of the bread followed by the eggs. Sprinkle heavy cream on top.

e. Cook in the oven for about 20 minutes. Once done, remove from the oven and garnish with remaining chives.

Nutritional Information:

Each serving contains 191 calories, 50 milligrams of calcium, 12 grams of fat, 2 milligrams of iron, 4 grams of saturated fat, 1 gram of fiber, 234 milligrams of cholesterol, 9 grams of carbohydrates, 426 milligrams of sodium and 12 milligrams of protein.

4. Goat Cheese Omelet with Herbs

Preparation Time: 5 minutes

Cook Time: 5 minutes

Number of Servings: 1

Ingredients:

3 eggs, beaten

2 oz. goat cheese, crumbled

1 tablespoon parsley, chopped

1 tablespoon butter, unsalted

1/8 teaspoon pepper black pepper

½ teaspoon kosher salt

Preparation:

a. Combine parsley and eggs together in a bowl. Season to taste.

b. Cook egg mixture in butter for about 4 minutes.

c. Distribute goat cheese over the eggs.

d. Fold the eggs in half and cook for another minute.

Nutritional Information:

Each serving contains 523 calories, 258 milligrams of calcium, 43 grams of fat, 4 milligrams of iron, 24 grams of saturated fat, 3 grams of sugar, 709 milligrams of cholesterol, 3 grams of carbohydrates, 1,466 milligrams of sodium and 31 grams of protein.

5. Scallion and Prosciutto Frittata

Preparation Time: 10 minutes

Cook Time: 20 minutes

Number of Servings: 4

Ingredients:

3 tablespoons extra virgin olive oil

4 oz. goat cheese, crumbled

6 scallions

¼ teaspoon kosher salt

4 oz. prosciutto, sliced thinly

4 cups arugula

8 eggs

¼ teaspoon black pepper

3 tablespoons whole milk

2 oz. parmesan cheese, grated

Preparation:
   a. Preheat oven to 350 degrees. Slice the scallions thinly on a diagonal direction and tear the prosciutto into 1-inch pieces.
   b. Cook the scallions in 1 tablespoon of olive oil for 1 ½ minutes.
   c. Add prosciutto and cook for another 4 minutes while stirring occasionally.
   d. Combine eggs, cheese, milk, and black pepper together in a bowl. Mix well.
   e. Transfer the egg mixture into the skillet and give everything a stir.
   f. Put the skillet in the oven and cook for about 20 minutes.
   g. Place equal amount of arugula in the plates. Sprinkle remaining olive oil and goat cheese on top. Season with salt.

h. Once cooked, slice the frittata and place it on top of the arugula salad.

Nutritional Information:

Each serving contains 441 calories, 1 gram of fiber, 34 grams of fat, 3 grams of sugar, 10 grams of saturated fat, 4 grams of carbohydrates, 464 milligrams of cholesterol, 31 grams of protein and 666 milligrams of sodium.

6. Scrambled Eggs with Spinach

Preparation Time: 5 minutes

Cook time: 5 minutes

Number of Servings: 4

Ingredients:

12 eggs, beaten

2 cups baby spinach

2 tablespoons olive oil

2 tablespoons Parmesan cheese, grated

2 scallions, chopped

½ cup cherry tomato, halved

1 tablespoon butter, cold

Black pepper, ground

Kosher salt

Preparation:

a. Saute scallions in oil for a minute.

b. Add butter and eggs. Cook while stirring.

c. Once cooked but creamy, put eggs in a plate. Add tomatoes, baby spinach and cheese. Mix well and season to taste.

Nutritional Information:

Each serving contains 325 calories, 147 milligrams of calcium, 26 grams of fat, 3 milligrams of iron, 8 grams of saturated fat, 1 gram of fiber, 645 milligrams of cholesterol, 2 grams of sugar, 534 milligrams of sodium, 4 grams of carbohydrates and 21 grams of sodium.

Chapter 3   - Seafood Dishes

1.   Poached Pacific Sole

Preparation Time: 10 minutes

Cook Time: 15 minutes

Number of Servings: 4

Ingredients:

¾ cup dry white wine

2 tablespoon chives, chopped

1 lb. sole fillets

2 tablespoons caper

2 tablespoons olive oil

1/8 teaspoon black pepper

¼ teaspoon kosher salt

Preparation:

a.   Pour wine into a skillet and warm it over medium heat.

b.   Slice the sole into spatula-size pieces and cook it in wine. Sprinkle olive oil, black pepper and salt over it.

c.   Add the capers. Cover the skillet and cook for another 4 minutes.

d.   Once the fish and capers are cooked through, place the chives on top.

Nutritional Information:

Each serving contains 189 calories, 20 grams of protein, 9 grams of fat, 504 milligrams of sodium, 1 gram of saturated fat, and 57 milligrams of cholesterol.

2. Shrimp with Horseradish Salsa

Preparation Time: 25 minutes

Cook Time: 5 minutes

Number of Servings: 4

Ingredients:

6 tablespoons lemon juice

2 heads Bibb lettuce

1 bay leaf

1 pint cherry tomatoes, halved

1 lb. shrimp, deveined and peeled

3 tablespoons extra-virgin olive oil

1 tablespoon prepared horseradish

¼ teaspoon kosher salt

8 cups water

2 ¼ teaspoon black pepper

Preparation:
   a. Remove the outer leaves of the Bibb lettuce and discard.
   b. Combine water, 3 tablespoons of lemon juice, bay leaf, lemon juice and 2 teaspoons of salt together in a large pot.
   c. Bring mixture to a boil then add shrimps. Cook for another 3 minutes.
   d. Transfer the shrimps to a bowl containing ice water. Once cooled, drain the shrimps and pat them dry.
   e. Place horseradish, remaining lemon juice and olive oil in a bowl and mix well. Season to taste.
   f. Add tomatoes and stir well. Serve on a bed of lettuce leaves and with salsa on top.

Nutritional Information:

Each serving contains 138 calories, 29 milligrams of calcium, 11 grams of fat, 1 milligrams of iron, 1 gram of saturated fat, 1 gram of fiber, 54 milligrams of cholesterol, 5 grams of carbohydrates, 149 milligrams of sodium and 7 milligrams of protein.

3. Baked Halibut

Preparation Time: 15 minutes

Cook Time: 10 minutes

Number of Servings: 4

Ingredients:

4 6-oz. halibut fillet, skinless

2 cups basil leaves

2 tablespoons olive oil

12 sprigs thyme

10. oz. spinach leaves

1 orange, sliced thin

¾ teaspoon kosher salt

½ teaspoon black pepper

Preparation:

a. Preheat oven to 400 degrees. Prepare four 15-inch parchment sheets.

b. Place the fish on one side of the parchment sheets. Season with half of the black pepper and ½ teaspoon of salt.

c. Distribute thyme and orange slices on top.

d. Cover each fish by folding the parchment sheet over it. Seal each sheet by folding the overlapping edges.

e. Place the parchment-covered fish fillets in 2 baking sheets.

f. Cook the fish in the oven for 12 minutes.

g. Saute spinach in oil over medium-high heat for about 3 minutes. Season to taste and sprinkle basil on top.

h. Serve the fish together with the cooked spinach leaves.

Nutritional Information:

Each serving contains 350 calories, 286 milligrams of calcium, 12 grams of fat, 5 milligrams of iron, 2 grams of saturated fat, 5 grams of fiber, 70 milligrams of cholesterol, 3 grams of sugar, 548 milligrams of sodium, 10 grams of carbohydrates and 50 grams of protein.

4. Salmon with Citrus

Preparation Time: 5 minutes

Cook Time 25 minutes

Number of Servings: 8

Ingredients:

3 lb. salmon fillet, skinless

12 sprigs thyme

1 tablespoon olive oil

1 lemon, sliced thinly

¾ teaspoon salt

1 orange, sliced thinly

½ teaspoon black pepper

Preparation:

a. Preheat oven to 375 degrees. Line a baking sheet with parchment paper.

b. Put the salmon in the prepared baking sheet and drizzle olive oil on top. Season with black pepper and salt.

c. Arrange lemon, orange, and thyme around the fish.

d. Cook the fish in the oven for about 25 minutes.

e. Once done, transfer the salmon in a plate. Distribute the citrus slices and thyme on top.

Nutritional Information:

Each serving contains 242 calories, 1 gram of fiber, 8 grams of fat, 2 grams of sugar, 1 gram of saturated fat, 3 grams of carbohydrates, 97 milligrams of cholesterol, 37 grams of protein and 305 milligrams of sodium.

Chapter 4 - Chicken Dishes

1. Pesto Chicken Salad

Preparation Time: 10 minutes

Cook Time: none

Number of Servings: 4

Ingredients:

½ cup mayonnaise

½ teaspoon salt

6 cups arugula

½ cup pesto

¼ teaspoon black pepper

2.5 lb. rotisserie chicken, chopped

Preparation:

a. Except for arugula, place all of the ingredients in a bowl and combine thoroughly.

b. Arrange arugula in a plate and place chicken salad on top.

Nutritional Information:

Each serving contains 627 calories, 290 milligrams of calcium, 47 grams of fat, 3 milligrams of iron, 10 grams of saturated fat, 3 milligrams of iron, 144 milligrams of cholesterol, 1 gram of fiber, 756 milligrams of sodium, 1 gram of sugar, 47 grams of protein and 3 grams of carbohydrates.

2. Grilled Chicken with Salad

Preparation Time: 5 minutes

Cook Time: 15 minutes

Number of Servings: 4

Ingredients:

3 tablespoons olive oil

½ red onion, sliced

4 6-oz. skinless chicken breasts, deboned

4 radishes, sliced

½ teaspoon coriander, ground

6 cups baby arugula

1 teaspoon salt

3 tablespoons lemon juice

½ teaspoon black pepper

Preparation:
a. Turn up grill to high.
b. Lean the grill gate and apply some oil to it.
c. Slice the chicken breasts horizontally and pound each piece to 1/2 –inch thickness.
d. Sprinkle coriander, half of the salt and half of the black pepper over the chicken slices. Cook each piece for about 3 minutes on the grill.
e. Combine lemon juice and olive oil together in a bowl. Season using remaining black pepper and salt.
f. Add remaining ingredients to the mixture and mix well.
g. Serve grilled chicken together with salad.

Nutritional Information:

Each serving contains 289 calories, 71 milligrams of calcium, 14 grams of fat, 2 milligrams of iron, 3 grams of saturated fat, 1 gram of fiber, 94 milligrams of cholesterol, 1 gram of sugar, 572 milligrams of sodium, 3 grams of carbohydrates and 35 grams of protein.

3. Braised Chicken with Vegetables

Preparation Time: 5 minutes

Cook Time: 30 minutes

Number of Servings: 4

Ingredients:

1 tablespoon olive oil

2 tablespoons chives, chopped

2.5 lb. chicken thighs

1 teaspoon sugar

½ teaspoon salt

4 carrots

¼ teaspoon black pepper

12 radishes, halved

1 cup chicken broth, low sodium

Preparation:
a. Slice the carrots into sticks. Sprinkle black pepper and salt over chicken.
b. Using a Dutch oven, cook chicken in oil over medium-high heat for 7 minutes on each side. Once done, place chicken in a plate.
c. Remove the fat from the pot and place it back in the heat.
d. Pour in the broth and scrape the bottom of the pot. Add radishes, sugar and carrots and place the chicken on top.
e. Cook gently for 20 minutes while partly covered. Garnish with chives.

Nutritional Information:

Each serving contains 237 calories, 47 milligrams of calcium, 13 grams of fat, 2 milligrams of iron, 3.5 grams of saturated fat, 2 grams of fiber, 100 milligrams of cholesterol, 5 grams of sugar, 426 milligrams of sodium, 9 grams of carbohydrates and 29 grams of protein.

Chapter 5 - Red Meat Dishes

1. Roasted Steak with Herbs

Preparation Time: 10 minutes

Cook time: 20 minutes

Number of Servings: 4

Ingredients:

¾ cup parsley, finely chopped

1 vidalia onion, peeled and sliced

2 cloves garlic, peeled and finely chopped

1.5 lb. skirt steak

1 ½ teaspoon oregano leaves, finely chopped

1/8 teaspoon black pepper, ground

3 tablespoons olive oil

¼ teaspoon kosher salt

1 tablespoon red wine vinegar

Preparation:

a. Place parsley, oregano, and garlic in a bowl. Drizzle with olive oil and season to taste. Mix well.

b. Preheat broiler. Slice the steak into 4 pieces.

c. Apply the herb mixture on both sides of each piece.

d. Broil steak for about 4 minutes on each side.

e. Once done, remove from heat and allow to rest for 5 minutes.

Nutrition Information:

Each serving contains 425 calories, 68 milligrams of calcium, 25 grams of fat, 6 milligrams of iron, 7 grams of saturated fat, 1 gram of fiber, 88 milligrams of cholesterol, 7 grams of carbohydrates, 272 milligrams of sodium and 41 milligrams of protein.

2. Pork Chops with Mustard Sauce

Preparation Time: 15 minutes

Cook time: 5 minutes

Number of Servings: 4

Ingredients:

3 tablespoons olive oil

8 lemon wedges

1.5 lb. pork chops, deboned

4 cups frisee, chopped

2 shallots, chopped

1 tablespoon tarragon, chopped

¾ cup dry white wine

1 tablespoon Dijon mustard

2 tablespoons heavy cream

½ teaspoon black pepper

½ teaspoon salt

Preparation:
   a. Preheat oven to 400 degrees.
   b. Slice pork chop into four 1-inch thick pieces. Season to taste.
   c. Cook pork chops in 1 tablespoon of olive oil over medium-high heat for 3 minutes on each side.
   d. Place pork chops on a baking sheet and allow to roast in the oven for 7 minutes. Once done, transfer them to a plate.
   e. In the meantime, saute shallots in 1 tablespoon of oil for about 4 minutes.
   f. Add white wine and bring it to a simmer.

g. Add cream once the wine is reduced by half. Cook the mixture gently until thick. Add mustard and stir well.

h. Drizzle the sauce over the pork chops. Sprinkle remaining olive oil over frisee ad serve together with lemon wedges.

Nutritional Information:

Each serving contains 364 calories, 2 grams of fiber, 19 grams of fat, 6 grams of carbohydrates, 6 grams of saturated fat, 37 grams of protein, 108 milligrams of cholesterol and 357 milligrams of sodium.

3. Lamb Chops with Tomatoes

Preparation Time: 5 minutes

Cook Time: 20 minutes

Number of Servings: 4

Ingredients:

1 tablespoon olive oil

¼ cup parsley

2 lb. lamb loin chops

¼ cup kalamata olives, pitted

1 teaspoon paprika

4 plum tomatoes, quartered

¼ teaspoon kosher salt

4 shallots, halved

½ teaspoon black pepper

Preparation:
a. Preheat oven to 400 degrees.
b. Slice lamb into 4 1 ½-inch thick pieces and season with salt, paprika, and black pepper.
c. Cook lamb in olive oil over medium-high heat for 3 minutes on each side.
d. Add shallots. Place lamb in the oven and cook for another 8 minutes.
e. Once done, place the lamb in plates.
f. Place olives, tomatoes and parsley in the skillet with lamb drippings. Toss everything to combine. Serve the vegetables with the lamb.

Nutritional Information:

Each serving contains 188 calories, 1 gram of fiber, 10 grams of fat, 3 grams of sugar, 2 grams of saturated fat, 9 grams of carbohydrates, 44 milligrams of cholesterol, 15 grams of protein and 544 milligrams of sodium.

4. Pork with Mustard Vinaigrette

Preparation Time: 5 minutes

Cook Time: 30 minutes

Number of Servings: 4

Ingredients:

1/3 cup extra virgin olive oil

1 tablespoon mustard, whole grain

1 pork tenderloin

2 tablespoons cider vinegar

½ teaspoon salt

3 shallots

½ teaspoon black pepper

1 lb. asparagus

Preparation:

a. Preheat oven to 400 degrees. Place vinegar, olive oil, and mustard in a bowl. Mix well and set aside.

b. Use ¼ teaspoon each of black pepper and salt to season the pork.

c. Cook the pork over medium heat for 3 minutes on each side.

d. Place the skillet in the oven and allow pork to roast for 15 minutes. Once done, set it aside to rest for 5 minutes.

e. Slice shallots into wedges and remove the tough ends of the asparagus. Place them in a rimmed baking sheet and drizzle some olive oil over them. Toss gently to coat and season with remaining black pepper and salt.

f. Place the vegetables in the oven and allow to roast for 15 minutes.

g. Once pork and vegetables are done, place them in a plate. Drizzle prepared mustard vinaigrette on top.

Nutritional Information:

Each serving contains 465 calories, 2 grams of fiber, 32 grams of fat, 4 grams of sugar, 6 grams of saturated fat, 8 grams of carbohydrates, 111 milligrams of cholesterol, 39 grams of protein and 332 milligrams of sodium.

Chapter 6 - Vegetarian Dishes

1. Broiled Asparagus

Preparation Time: 4 minutes

Cook Time: 10 minutes

Number of Servings: 4

Ingredients:

1 lb. asparagus, trimmed

¼ teaspoon salt

2 tablespoons olive oil

¼ teaspoon black pepper

Preparation:

a. Preheat broiler. Place asparagus in a single layer on a baking sheet and drizzle with olive oil. Season to taste.

b. Place the baking sheet in the broiler and allow to cook for 8 minutes. Make sure to shake the baking sheet occasionally.

c. Once tender, transfer the asparagus in a plate. Serve with grated Parmesan cheese or crumbled feta cheese if desired.

Nutritional Information:

Each serving contains 88 calories, 2 grams of fiber, 7 grams of fat, 2 grams of sugar, 1 gram of saturated fat, 4 grams of carbohydrates, 122 milligrams of sodium and 3 grams of protein.

2. No-Meat Burger

Preparation Time: 10 minutes

Cook Time: 10 minutes

Number of Servings: 6

Ingredients:

6 tomatoes, halved

2 sprigs basil leaves

2 tablespoons olive oil

8 oz. mozzarella, unsalted

1 teaspoon kosher salt

1 clove garlic, sliced thinly

¼ teaspoon black pepper

Preparation:

a. Preheat oven to 450 degrees. Line a rimmed baking sheet with aluminium foil.

b. Place the tomato slices on the prepared baking sheet with the cut-side up.

c. Sprinkle olive oil over tomatoes and season to taste. Distribute garlic on top.

d. Place the baking sheet in the oven and allow tomatoes to roast for 15 minutes.

e. Slice mozzarella into 6 pieces that are ½-inch thick.

f. Assemble your burger by placing the mozzarella slices in between two tomato pieces.

g. Sprinkle the burgers with cooking juices from the pan. Garnish with basil.

Nutritional Information:

Each serving contains 182.15 calories, 21.52 milligrams of calcium, 12.98 grams of fat, 0.59 milligrams of iron, 6.08 grams of saturated fat, 2.26 grams of fiber, 29.7 milligrams of cholesterol, 8.32 grams of carbohydrates, 196.11 milligrams of sodium and 8.43 milligrams of protein.

3. Arugula Salad with Radishes

Preparation Time: 10 minutes

Cook time: none

Number of Servings: 4

Ingredients:

6 cups arugula

8 tablespoons creamy parmesan dressing

1 bulb fennel, cored and sliced thinly

6 radishes

4 oz. green beans, sliced

Preparation:

a. Slice the radishes into wedges.

b. Place the radish wedges in a bowl together with the remaining ingredients and toss to coat.

Nutritional Information:

Each serving contains 134 calories, 152 milligrams of calcium, 10 grams of fat, 1 milligram of iron, 2 grams of saturated fat, 3 grams of fiber, 6 milligrams of cholesterol, 1 gram of sugar, 155 milligrams of sodium, 8 grams of carbohydrates and 4 grams of protein.

4. Lettuce and Citrus Salad

Preparation Time: 20 minutes

Cook Time: none

Number of Servings: 8

Ingredients:

3 heads Boston lettuce, torn

¼ teaspoon black pepper

2 navel oranges, peeled and sliced thinly

½ teaspoon kosher salt

1 tablespoon white wine vinegar

¾ cup pecans, toasted and chopped

¼ cup extra virgin olive oil

4 oz. goat cheese, crumbled

1 shallot, minced

¼ cup orange juice

Preparation:

a. Place orange juice, black pepper, olive oil, vinegar, salt, and shallot in a bowl. Mix well.

b. Combine the remaining ingredients together in a bowl. Drizzle prepared dressing over the salad and toss to coat.

Nutritional Information:

Each serving contains 159.85 calories, 45.13 milligrams of calcium, 14.25 grams of fat, 1.15 milligrams of iron, 1.56 grams of saturated fat, 2.46 grams of fiber, 73.87 milligrams of sodium, 8 grams of carbohydrates and 2.17 milligrams of protein.

Chapter 7 - Snacks and Desserts

1. Zucchini Chips

Preparation Time: 10 minutes

Cook Time: 10 minutes

Number of Servings: 4

Ingredients:

2 zucchinis

2 tablespoons parmesan cheese, grated

2 tablespoons extra virgin olive oil

¼ teaspoon black pepper

¼ teaspoon salt

Preparation:

a. Turn up your oven to 400 degrees.

b. Slice zucchini into ¼-inch strips.

c. Coat zucchini strips in olive oil and cheese. Season to taste.

d. Arrange the zucchini strips in a single layer on a baking sheet and place them in the oven.

e. Bake for 10 minutes. Turn them once hallway through the cook.

f. Once done, transfer them into a wire rack to cool.

Nutritional Information:

Each serving contains 2.2 grams of protein, 0.9 grams of fiber, 8 grams of fat, 88 calories and 2.3 grams of net carbohydrates.

2. Creamy Berry Tarts

Preparation Time: 15 minutes

Cook Time: 10 minutes

Number of Servings: 4

Ingredients:

2/3 cups almonds, slivered and chopped

¼ cup heavy cream

½ cup raspberries

½ cup blueberries

2 tablespoons Sucralose based sweetener

Preparation:

a. Preheat broiler.

b. Place equal amounts of almonds in 4 ramekins and sprinkle half of the sweetener on top of each.

c. Arrange the ramekins in a cookie sheet and put it in the broiler.

d. Once sweetener has melted, remove from heat and set aside to cool.

e. Combine remaining sweetener and heavy cream together in a bowl. Whisk until the cream has doubled in volume.

f. Distribute the raspberries and blueberries equally among the ramekins. Put whipped cream on top.

Nutritional Information:

Each serving contains 4.5 grams of protein, 3.6 grams of fiber, 14.6 grams of fat, 177 calories and 6 grams of net carbohydrates.

3. Vanilla Mousse with Rhubarb Sauce

Preparation Time: 15 minutes

Cook Time: 10 minutes

Number of Servings: 2

Ingredients:

2 stalks rhubarb

½ cup heavy cream

3 teaspoons Sucralose based sweetener

¼ cup water

4 oz. Greek yogurt, plain

1 tablespoon strawberry jam, sugar free

Preparation:

a. Place the water, rhubarb and strawberry jam in a saucepan. Mix well and cook over medium heat.

b. Once simmering, turn down the heat to medium low and secure the lid.

c. Cook gently for about 10 minutes while stirring occasionally. Allow to cool.

d. Combine remaining ingredients together in a bowl. Whisk the mixture using an electric mixer on medium-high speed until semi-firm peaks form.

e. Spread ¼ cup of vanilla mousse evenly in the bottom of a glass. Drizzle 1 ½ tablespoons of rhubarb sauce over it.

f. Repeat procedure using a second glass.

g. Continue dividing the remaining ingredients between the two glasses until everything have been used up.

Nutritional Information:

Each serving contains 5.4 grams of protein, 0.9 grams of fiber, 28 grams of fat, 301 calories and 8.1 grams of net carbohydrates.

4. Mascarpone Parfait

Preparation Time: 15 minutes

Cook Time: none

Number of Servings: 4

Ingredients:

1 cup heavy cream

1 tablespoon Sucralose based sweetener

8 oz. mascarpone

Preparation:

a. Whisk heavy cream using an electric mixer on medium-high speed.

b. Once soft peaks form, turn down the speed to medium.

c. Add sweetener and mascarpone. Continue whisking for 30 seconds.

d. Distribute cream mixture among four parfait cups.

Nutritional Information:

Each serving contains 5.3 grams of protein, 48.5 grams of fat, 451 calories and 2 grams of net carbohydrates.

5. Coconut Cookies

Preparation Time: 8 minutes

Cook Time: 27 minutes

Number of Servings: 12

Ingredients:

½ cup whole grain soy flour

7 tablespoons Sucralose based sweetener

1/3 cup coconut, dried

8 tablespoons butter, unsalted

¼ cup whole hazelnuts, toasted and chopped

½ teaspoon salt

1 ½ teaspoons coconut extract

2 egg whites

½ teaspoon vanilla extract

1/8 can seltzer water

Preparation:

a. Turn up oven to 375 degrees. Use non-stick cooking spray to grease a baking sheet.

b. Combine all of the ingredients together in a bowl and mix well.

c. Form 12 equal-sized balls from the mixture and place them on the baking sheet. Lightly press each ball to flatten them slightly.

d. Cook in the oven for 20 minutes. Once done, allow to cool for a minute before transferring them in a wire rack.

Nutritional Information:

Each serving contains 2.8 grams of protein, 1.3 grams of fiber, 12.4 grams of fat, 134 calories and 2.2 grams of net carbohydrates.

6. Pistachio Butter Cookies

Preparation Time: 20 minutes

Cook Time: 16 minutes

Number of Servings: 24

Ingredients:

1/8 teaspoon salt

1 teaspoon vanilla extract

1/3 cup sucralose based sweetener

1 cup oatmeal, dry

½ cup pistachio nuts, roasted and unsalted

1/3 cup whole grain wheat flour

½ cup butter, unsalted

1/3 cup whole grain soy flour

1 egg

¼ teaspoon straight phosphate baking powder, double acting

Preparation:

a. Turn up oven to 375 degrees. Use a non-stick cooking spray to grease a baking sheet.

b. Place pistachio, baking powder, oatmeal, salt, sweetener, soy flour and wheat flour in a food processor. Pulse for about 1 minute.

c. Add egg and butter and pulse mixture for 15 seconds.

d. Place the dough in the refrigerator for 15 minutes.

e. Form 24 equal-sized dough balls and arrange them in the prepared baking sheet. Lightly press on each ball to flatten them slightly.

f. Cook the cookies in the oven for 16 minutes. Allow to cool for a minute before transferring to a wire rack.

Nutritional Information:

Each serving contains 1.5 grams of protein, 0.6 grams of fiber, 5.5 grams of fat, 66 calories and 2.5 grams of net carbohydrates.

Conclusion...Call to action!

Thank you again for downloading this book!

I hope this book was able to help you achieve your weight loss goals with these healthy, low carb recipes.

A low carb diet allows you to enjoy a variety of food products while helping you lose weight and stay healthy. In addition, you wouldn't find difficulty sticking to this diet because you wouldn't feel deprived. It can also help you reduce your food intake naturally by making you feel sated for a longer period of time.

The next step is to make your low carb diet a lifetime food regimen to stay healthy.

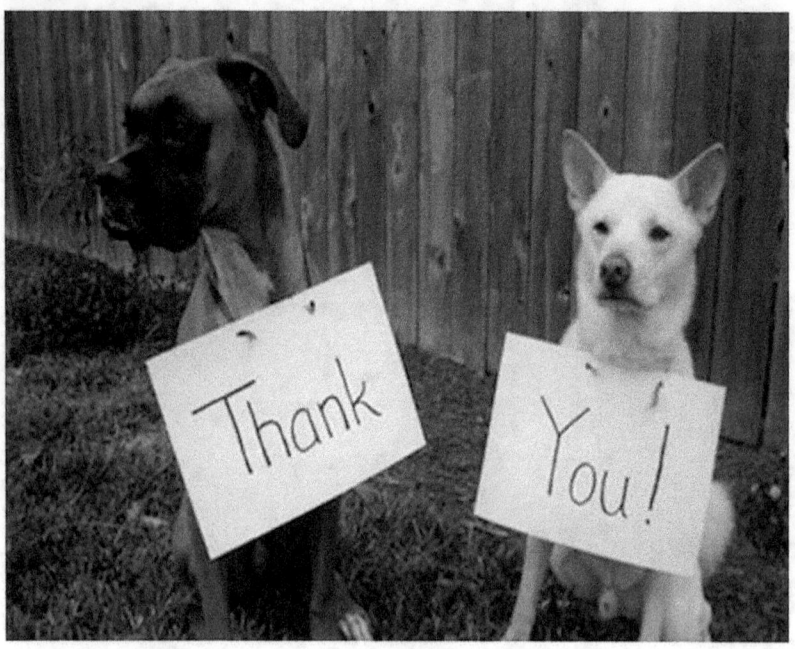

Finally, if you enjoyed this book, then I'd like to ask you for a favor, would you be kind enough to leave a review for this book on Amazon? It'd be greatly appreciated!

Click here to leave a review for this book on Amazon!

Thank you and good luck!

Below you'll find some of my other popular books that are popular on Amazon and Kindle as well. Simply click on the links below to check them out. Alternatively, you can visit my author page on Amazon to see other work done by me.

<u>My Other Book - This Is My Other Book On Amazon</u>

FREE BONUS CLICK LINK

www.ingramcontent.com/pod-product-compliance
Lightning Source LLC
Chambersburg PA
CBHW071254280526
45788CB00004B/1712